Weight Lifting for Body Sculpting

Build Your Dream Body thru Weight Lifting

By Kevin Whiting

I0427869

Table of Contents

Introduction

I want to thank you and congratulate you for downloading the book, *"Weight Lifting for Body Sculpting: Build Your Dream Body thru Weight Lifting"*.

This book contains proven steps and strategies on how to sculpt your entire body using different weight training techniques.

Weight Lifting for Body Sculpting is a book that's designed to help you create the body of your dreams thru various weight training exercises. This book will teach you some of the best muscle-building workouts that utilize weight training equipment such as dumbbells, barbells, and machines. It is a sure-fire guide to have that ripped physique without resorting to illegal and potentially hazardous substances. We'll teach you how to pump iron right and gain mass and strength the effective and safe way.

Thanks again for downloading this book, I hope you enjoy it!

Chapter 1: Why Weight Lifting?

Physical conditioning is power, both literally and figuratively. When you are in top shape, you can perform at the highest level your body can achieve while at the same time reducing the potential of developing injuries, illnesses, and other physical ailments. There are many forms of physical conditioning techniques developed and one of the most applied and most versatile of them all is weight lifting. Why exactly should you go for weight training?

The first evidence of the concept of resistance training was seen on ancient Greece. The Greeks, who are notoriously fascinated with both their looks and physical abilities, are known to lift heavy objects both for show and for improving their physique. The legendary Greek doctor Galen also described exercises that utilize halters, a primitive form of the dumbbell. It is during the 19th century when the concept of weight lifting for fitness has been established. Common weight training tools such as the dumbbell, barbell, kettlebell, and clubbell were developed and utilized extensively during this time. By the time the 20th century rolled around, machines are created to complement these free-weight exercise tools. By the 1960s, during the fitness boom, gyms became very popular, bringing weight lifting closer to the masses.

While everyone is doing it, you might still doubt why you should utilize weight training as your means to sculpt and fine-tune your body. Here are some of the most compelling benefits of weight lifting for health.

1. Increased muscle mass- Muscles are known to be developed with both resistance and continuous stimulation. When muscles are commonly used and regularly subjected to strenuous activity, they compensate by increasing in mass (hypertrophy) and increasing in number (hyperplasia). Both

physiological conditions bring about the expansion of muscles, and with it come the physical rewards of weight training such as increased mass, strength, and endurance.

2. Enhanced body composition- It is one thing that muscle mass is significantly improved by weight lifting. Constant weight training is known to trim off fat as it does use off calories. Also, it causes a physiological shift that prevents lean body mass loss during a caloric deficit. Last but not least, engaging in physical activity such as these improves bone mass, preventing conditions such as osteoporosis from taking over and breaking the bones.

3. Better metabolism- Constant weight training can significantly increase your metabolism. This is because muscle tissue consumes the most energy among all tissues per unit mass. Developing muscle thru weight lifting increases basal metabolic rate, the speed in which you burn calories while you're at rest. The benefits of better metabolism are numerous. It promotes long-term fat loss, and it also stabilizes your eating habits.

4. Improved appearance- The reason why people go for weight training is to improve their looks. After all, who doesn't want to have a muscular and toned physique? A body that's sculpted by proper weight training methods is considered attractive. Both men and women can benefit from weight training in the looks department, and it can help them improve both their self-confidence and level of approval from others.

5. Increased performance- Constant weight lifting is seen to improve physical abilities a lot. Measurable athletic traits such as strength, speed, jumping ability, endurance, and explosiveness can all be improved by using the right weight training techniques. Traditionally, weight training is only used for strength-based sports such as bodybuilding, weightlifting, shotput, and javelin throw, but it's now widely used as a conditioning tool for other sports ranging from track and field to combat sports.

Chapter 2: Building Up Your Chest

The chest is one of the most prominent muscles in your entire body. It is mainly composed of 2 muscle groups: the pectoralis major and the pectoralis minor. The pectoralis major is the fleshy muscle you most observe protruding in your chest. Mainly originating from the ribs and sternum area and inserting into the arms and shoulders, the chest, also known as the "pecs", have very particular functions. The pectoralis major is responsible for lifting the arms from the front and side, as well as turning the arm in an arm-wrestling motion. The pectoralis minor's main function is to stabilize the scapula, a bone that connects the upper arm (humerus) and the collar bone (clavicle).

There are tangible benefits in shaping up your chest. It is already given that since it's one of the major muscles in the body, it's bound to be seen by others. In short, a well-toned chest is considered attractive for both sexes. It also improves your arm strength significantly, especially when it comes to lifting, pushing, swinging, and throwing motions. Last but not least, it helps in stabilizing the arms and shoulders, reducing the risk of injuries on that region.

Here is a list of some of the must-try weight training exercises for your chest.

1. Bench press- The bench press is one of the most basic weight lifting exercises in the book. An effective form of compound exercise, it is an effective means of measuring and improving overall upper body strength. Can be performed using a barbell or a pair of equally-weighted dumbbells, not only does it effectively build up the chest muscles, but it also attacks the muscles of the arms and shoulders. It also works on the stabilizing muscles located near the chest, shoulders,

and core. Adjusting bench angle allows you to attack particular muscle regions.

2. Pushup- The pushup is another favorite for fitness junkies around the world. Another effective form of compound exercise, it uses the person's own weight as a source of resistance. Hand positioning is one great way to vary which muscle groups are stimulated by the pushup. According to studies, doing close-gripped pushups (narrower than the shoulders) stimulate the chest best. The best thing about the pushup is that it's something you can do anywhere without the need for special equipment.

3. Cable crossovers- Crossovers are an effective way of working on your chest muscles. This routine takes advantage of the benefits provided by cable machines, most particularly providing consistent tension in all ranges of motion. Crossover 21s is a great way to attack the chest from all angles. At the low position, pull the cable up to eye level. At the middle position, pull the cable forward until both your arms touch each other. At the high position, press the handles down to in front of your abdomen. Perform 7 reps at each position to complete a set (7 x 3 = 21, hence the name 21s).

4. Forward-leaning dips- The dip is a killer exercise that's physically demanding. This would provide a great challenge for experienced fitness junkies. While most dips are done at an upright position (hence targeting the arms first), it can become a devastating chest-building exercise by leaning your forward during execution. Because of the degree of difficulty of this exercise, this is best done with a spotter to keep your body balanced. If you have a history of shoulder injuries, start off on a small range of motion to determine how deep you can go.

Chapter 3: Strengthening Your Back

A strong back is essential for optimal physical health. This region is composed of massive muscles that provide stability for both your spine and core, 2 regions that are integral for maintaining structural integrity in your body. Because of the sheer size of the back, it contains all kinds of muscles. They include the lattismus dorsi (lats), erector spinae (erectors), trapezius (traps), teres major and minor, and rhomboid major and minor.

The benefits of keeping your back muscles strong are numerous, and each of these benefits can help you out no matter what your age, gender, or fitness level. First, it keeps your spine strong and flexible, essential for preventing both back pain and spinal issues. Also, it helps in keeping your body stable, essential for maintaining proper posture both while stationary and during movement. In case you don't know, your posture can either prevent or increase your risk of injury, especially on weight bearing joints. Lastly, strong back muscles add more force to your movements, improving overall strength on the process.

Here are some exercises you can use to build the different muscles of your back. Over time, these can help you build a back that can take all kinds of punishment and will take people's collective breaths away.

1. Deadlift- The deadlift is another of those basic strength-testing exercises. While there are different forms of this explosive exercise, they all work on just about every critical muscle in your back. At the same time, it also stimulates the muscles of your core, shoulders, and legs. No matter what style you use, make sure that when executing deadlifts, you must keep your back straight while lifting to prevent injuries. When

done right, it's the best exercise to build big, strong, and powerful back muscles.

2. Rows- The row can be done while seated or while bent over. This can be performed using free weights such as dumbbells or using machines such as the cable. This exercise mainly targets the middle region of your back while also providing a good workout for your arms and back. While keeping your head up and your back straight, bend your arms over, pulling the weight towards your torso on the process. You shall feel your shoulder blades squeeze together during execution, which is a sign that you're stimulating your back muscles perfectly.

3. Pull-ups- The pull-up is one of the most punishing body weight exercises around. At the same time, it is a sure-fire way to create a powerful back. It targets just about every major back muscle, but it works the lats out the most. To perform this exercise, you'll grip on something located overhead (most commonly a bar). Using the sheer force of your upper body, lift your body up the bar until your chin is level with the bar. Swinging and kipping using your legs is not allowed as it adds extra momentum.

4. Back extension- This is one of the best ways to stimulate the muscles of your lower back, which is one of the most notoriously injury-prone regions of the human body. This exercise mainly stimulates the extensor muscles located at the middle portion of the back, which is essential for extending the lower back and turning it sideways. To perform this, you must lie with your face down. Resisting movement from your hips and legs, lift your torso by contracting your back muscles. Come back down smoothly to complete one rep.

Chapter 4: Powering Up Your Legs

Developing your lower body strength is very important for your physical well-being. You'll need to build up the strength of your lower limbs in order to perform a lot of your daily functions (especially movement-related) properly and effectively. Both the upper part (thigh) and the lower part (leg) of your limbs must be trained in order to bring out maximum lower body strength. The thigh is composed of muscles such as the quadriceps and the triceps femoris. The leg is composed of a few muscles, with the most prominent one being the gastrocnemius (calf).

Building your legs is very important in a lot of levels. In fact, it's laughable that most bodybuilders ignore the role of lower body strength in their day-to-day endeavors. Having strong legs mean that you'll gain better athletic performance related to using the legs (ex: running speed, jumping height). Also, the presence of strong muscles in the legs helps in carrying the weight of the body, making it much easier to move around. Last but not least, stronger leg muscles help in preventing injuries on weight-bearing bones/joints such as the knees and feet.

If you haven't been giving proper attention to your legs, it is time for you to do so now. Here are just some of the best exercises you can try to build both your thighs and legs.

1. Squats- This exercise is considered to be the quintessential exercise for developing big and strong thighs. It targets muscles such as the buttocks, quadriceps, and hamstrings. You can do this as a body weight exercise, but you can also use weights such as dumbbells and barbells to add resistance. To perform this, you must position yourself with your legs slightly apart. Lower your body until your thighs is parallel to the floor. Lift your body up using your legs to complete a rep.

Make sure to keep your back straight at all times when performing this exercise.

2. Leg press- You can do this exercise with the help of a leg press machine. First, determine how much weight to put into the machine (as a rule of thumb, it should be equal on the weight you do your squats). Sit on the machine with your back straight and position your feet shoulder width apart into the platform. Remove the lock and let the platform lower until your legs form a 90-degree angle. Then, push the platform up by straightening your legs. You can perform as many reps as you like. Just remember that before getting off the machine, you should secure the lock to prevent the platform from falling on you.

3. Lunges- The lunge is one of the best ways to build both your thighs and buttocks. You can perform this as a body weight exercise, or you can use weights to add more resistance to your training. Keep your back and shoulders straight and engage your core to keep your upper body stable. Step forward with one leg and lower your hips so that both knees form a 90-degree angle. Lift your body up to complete a rep. Perform lunges using both of your legs.

4. Calf raise- The calf raise is the main way to develop your calf muscle. This can be performed one-legged or two-legged, and can also be performed as a body weight exercise or with weights. If you're performing a two-legged calf raise, keep both feet on the ground at equal length. If you're performing a one-legged raise, lift the non-working leg up by bending your knee backwards. Lift your body by bending your toes. After that's done, slowly bring your body down to starting position. You can either do multiple reps of the calf raise, or you can try to hold your body up as long as you can.

Chapter 5: Ripping Up Your Arms

Having strong arms is a great indicator that you're putting in the extra work at the gym. Also, they are mostly exposed, so muscles from this region are easily exposed for all to see. Having toned, strong, and powerful arms definitely looks good, especially for men. The muscles of the upper arm (triceps and biceps) are primarily there to control the motion of the forearm. The muscles of the forearm mainly serve to control the hands and wrists.

The benefits of having a strong arm are numerous. First, it helps you lift heavier loads, especially when your back and shoulders are at prime condition. Second, it makes your grip stronger, which is essential for a lot of our everyday activities. Third, it helps us in pushing and pulling objects such as doors with ease. We use our arms extensively everyday, so it seems perfectly logical to make the effort in building its strength up.

The following is a list of some of the best weight training workouts you can use to build your arms. Follow these and you'll have strong, evenly proportioned, and properly toned arm muscles.

1. Bicep curls- The bicep curl is the most basic way to develop your biceps. You can perform this exercise either with a pair of dumbbells or kettelbells or a barbell. At the starting position, you must have your shoulders squared, back straight, feet shoulder apart, and the weights held by both hands with palms on front. To start the rep, flex your elbow until the weight is at chest/shoulder level, keeping excess movement at a minimum. Lower the weight to starting position to compete one rep. You can perform 10-15 reps per set or until muscle fatigue ensues.

2. Bench dips- The bench dip is an effective exercise for building the triceps. It uses your own body weight to provide resistance, and it would burn off the fat on the back of your

arms in no time. You'll need to place a bench behind you back. While looking away from it, hold on to the edge of the bench with both hands. Your hands must be straight and at shoulder width apart. Lower your body by bending your elbows until you are close to a 90-degree angle. After that, you must raise your body back to starting position using your arms. The number of reps you can do depends on your physical condition.

3. Triceps extension- This is essentially the opposite of the biceps curl. As the name would suggest, this exercise mainly targets the triceps. Just like the biceps curl, you can perform this exercise with the help of a dumbbell, a kettlebell, or a barbell. Position the weight overhead, making sure that your arm/s have a stable hold on the weight at all times. Lower your forearm together with the weight by flexing your elbows, careful not to hit your head with the weight. Raise the weight by extending your elbows. As a good starting point, use the same amount of resistance and reps that you use for your biceps curl.

4. Wrist curls- A lot of people ignore the importance of the forearm muscles. You'll need to build your forearms too for maximum effectiveness. Not only does it ensure that your arms remain proportional, but also to ensure maximum hand/wrist strength. With your forearms parallel to the floor, grab a dumbbell or a kettlebell like you would for a biceps curl. However, instead of flexing your elbows, you got to flex your wrists for lifting the weight. You can use either the supinated or pronated grip to target different forearm muscles.

Chapter 6: Broadening the Shoulders

The shoulder is responsible for connecting your arms to your torso. As this is a region subjected to high levels of stress, strengthening the muscles that surround the shoulder joint can be very beneficial for both strength development and injury prevention. There are a number of muscles located here, and their functions can range anywhere from rotating the arm to lifting the arm in multiple directions. Prominent muscles located at the shoulder include the deltoid, the trapezius, the teres muscles, and the supraspinatus.

So what are the benefits of developing your shoulders? First, because it is such a huge muscle region, developing your shoulders has a big impact on determining your overall upper body strength. Second, having broad, trim shoulders is a sure-fire way to look more attractive, regardless if you are a man or a woman. Third, it helps you avoid arm injuries, as the shoulder joint can be subjected to high amounts of stress every day.

Now that you know the importance of broadening those shoulders, it is now time to learn about the routines that will help you accomplish exactly that.

1. Military press- This exercise is great because it builds multiple shoulder muscles including the deltoids and trapezius. It also helps in improving arm, leg and core strength as they help in stabilizing your body as you lift. To perform this exercise, you'll need a barbell. At the starting point, the barbell should be at shoulder level. Both feet should be together and the back must remain straight. To execute the press, you should lift the barbell overhead by pressing it upwards. After the lift, you should go back to starting position to complete one rep.

2. Lateral/front raise- The front raise mainly targets the front end of the deltoids, while the lateral raise targets the middle. As such, both exercises can be used in the same workout for maximum gains in shoulder mass and strength. To perform the front raise, you got to hold a pair of dumbbells or kettlebells on both hands. Slowly lift your arms forward up to shoulder level, and then bring it down slowly. To perform the lateral raise, begin at the same starting position as the front raise. Lift your arms to the side until it is at shoulder level, and then bring it down slowly. Use both exercises to get strong deltoids.

3. External/internal rotations- This exercise is mainly designed to develop the rotator cuff, a group of muscles and tendons that stabilizes the shoulders. Muscles included in the rotator cuff include the teres minor, infraspinatus, supraspinatus, and the subscapularis. The starting position for this exercise is to hold a weight or the handle of a cable with your elbow bent at a 90-degree angle. Keeping your elbow bent, rotate your shoulder, bringing either your forearm inward or outward. Perform 12-16 reps of this exercise to complete a set.

4. Upright rows- Upright rows is one of the best exercises around if you want a compound exercise that would develop your shoulders. Not only does it target the shoulder muscles, but it also targets the upper back and the arms. To perform this exercise, you can use either a dumbbell or a barbell as your source of resistance. To start, hold the weight with your palms facing you. Bend your elbows and pull the weight upwards until it's at least on chest level. You can use different hand positions to target different muscle groups. For a more shoulder-centered workout, try to do this exercise with your hand farther apart.

Chapter 7: Make Your Core Hardcore

When you think about the core, the first thing that you think about is the abs. Well, that is true, the abdominal muscles are one of the most critical parts of the core, but it would sell it short to consider it as the only part of the core. Regardless, you can build your core and sculpt your body with the help of particular weight training exercises. By sharpening up your core, you can get all kinds of benefits that translate to a better physique and physical health.

There are many benefits associated with improving your core's conditioning. First, it improves your body's overall build as it helps you get rid of the nasty flab around your belly. Second, having a trim core aids in lowering your body's center of gravity, aiding in all kinds of biomechanical factors ranging from maintaining balance to making explosive movements. Third, it reduces the pressure from your back and hips, reducing the risk of injury in these major weight-bearing regions. Last but not least, having a strong core translates to better overall strength and endurance for all physical/athletic activity.

With the help of some weight training methods, you can get the strong, trim core you've wanted for so long. Even better is that you can get this faster than you ever think possible.

1. Windmills- This exercise is not just great for developing abs, but it is also awesome for toning those love handles. To begin, stand at a wide stance with your knees slightly bent. Hold a dumbbell with both hands to your chest at the starting position. To execute, rotate your torso using your abs, lifting the weight upwards using one arm. Return back to starting position to complete a rep. Make sure to perform the windmill exercise with equal reps on both sides. To add resistance, you can increase the weight or number of reps.

2. Vertical climbs- This exercise is not just great for working your core, but it can also provide an adequate workout for your

arms and legs. To perform this exercise, you'll need a pair of dumbbells. At the starting position, lift overhead one of the dumbbells. Then, as you lower down the raised arm, raise the opposite arm and raise the knee on the same side of the raised arm during the starting position. Return to starting position afterwards. Perform this exercise with both legs so that both sides of your core is stimulated.

3. Straight-arm climb- The straight-arm climb is a great alternative for the legendary crunches, especially if you're the type who's prone to back injuries. It's a seemingly harmless exercise, but a straight-arm climb can bust those ab muscles very effectively. To perform this, first lay down with your face up while holding 2 equal-weighted dumbbells straight up. Lift your head and neck off the floor, and alternately raise your left and right shoulder blades, respectively. 20 reps should be your baseline goal for each set.

4. Russian twists- The Russian twist is one of the most old-school ways in building a strong core. This exercise works the abdomen by performing a twisting motion, forcing the abdominal muscles to contract and support the body. To perform the Russian twist, sit on the floor with knees bent as if you'll be performing sit-ups. With weight in hand, raise your torso up at a 45-degree angle. The arms should be swung from side to side, with the abs keeping the entire body stable until the set is complete. You can make the swinging motion slower to increase the intensity of the workout.

Chapter 8: Extra Tips to Make It All Work

Lifting weights is just one step to creating the body of your dreams. In fact, there are more things you should do to ensure that you get the physique you always desire. A lot of people forget these and end up not getting that ripped body even while spending hours at the gym. There is more to building your body than just pumping iron. Here are some tips to ensure that you'll get the body of your dreams and make it stick for the long run.

1. Put emphasis on your diet- Bodybuilding experts, dieticians, and conditioning coaches all agree that your diet matters more than your workouts. Your management (or lack of it) of your diet has a huge say on how your body will eventually take shape. You got to regulate your calories so you won't deposit excess fat that can conceal your muscles. Still, you got to get enough nutrients to build muscle and keep bodily functions rolling.

2. Do some cardio exercises- Cardio is just as important when trying to build an imposing physique. While it offers only minimal benefits in terms of building and toning muscle, what it does it helps in burning off excess fat thru aerobic activity. At the same time, regular cardio increases a person's endurance so they can do more exercises per session. Some examples of cardio exercises include running, cycling, swimming, dance, interval training, and some sports.

3. Manage stress- One reason why your body is not taking shape like it should is because of stress. Stress is known to have a negative effect to one's body. First, it hampers metabolism, making it much easier for the body to store fat. Second, it alters one's food cravings, making people eat more than what they would usually eat. Last but not least, it causes the production of cortisol, which stimulates fat storage on the

body, particularly on the belly. Manage everyday stress and go one step closer to a fitter body.

4. Get enough rest- Having enough rest is very important in a number of ways. Getting sufficient rest is a great way to reduce stress and get your body ready for the next day. You'll need to incorporate rest days on your daily workout routine because that is the time when your muscles heal and rebuild themselves. Not getting enough rest has 2 negative impacts: it causes the eventual atrophy of muscles and it increases the risk of developing injuries.

5. Stay motivated- Having constant motivation is important to keep yourself going. There are 2 critical points in your journey that can shake your motivation and end up setting you back: failure and success. You got to understand that failure is part of the game and part of the challenge is how you'll actually respond to adversity. As for success, you got to find ways to keep your desire burning even after you've accomplished your fitness goals. It's best to make personal well-being your ultimate goal rather than making it about six-packs and lost pounds.

Conclusion

Thank you again for downloading this book!

I hope this book was able to help you to build your body thru weight training.

The next step is to apply the various tips in this book to shape all parts of your body. Follow them, stay the course, and you'll have your dream physique in no time!

Finally, if you enjoyed this book, please take the time to share your thoughts and post a review on Amazon. It'd be greatly appreciated!

Thank you and good luck!

Unlisted Bonus - Grain Free Recipes

Grains are generally classified as either cereals or legumes. Being an essential part of a normal diet, they provide not only carbohydrates but also numerous other nutrients such as fiber, antioxidants, iron and zinc. However, a percentage of today's generation chooses not to engage in this diet. Whatever reasons these people have, it is necessary for them to pursue a diet plan that does not include any product with grains.

Grain free Recipes are usually related to the Paleolithic diet – a nutritional plan that got its name from the lifestyle of humans in the Paleolithic period. This diet consists mainly of seafood, fruits and vegetables, eggs and other food that do not contain grains, legumes and a few processed items. Looking for **Grain free Recipes**, however, is becoming a challenge in today's society. Obvious enough, a big percentage of this generation's produce comes from grains.

This recipe is among numerous **Grain free Recipes** that dieters can try. It is a simple procedure for those who wish to pursue with this kind of diet, or even for those who just want to cut down on their grain intake.

The following ingredients are needed to make this recipe. These ingredients are also usually present in other **Grain free Recipes**.

- ✓ 1/2 teaspoon of salt
- ✓ 1 teaspoon of nutmeg
- ✓ 1 tablespoon of cinnamon
- ✓ 1/4 cup of powdered maca root
- ✓ 2/3 cup of melted coconut oil
- ✓ 3/4 cup of dried currants
- ✓ 3/4 cup of honey or maple syrup
- ✓ 1 cup of sesame seeds
- ✓ 1 and 1/2 cups of ground flax seed
- ✓ 2 cups of raw, unsalted pumpkin seeds
- ✓ 2 cups of raw, unsalted sunflower seeds

The following utensils and appliances are needed as well. Like ingredients, these utensils may also be required in making other **Grain free Recipes**.

- ✓ baking sheet
- ✓ parchment paper
- ✓ small and large bowls
- ✓ oven

The following a step-by-step procedure in making one of the several **Grain free Recipes** should be properly followed.

1. Adjust the oven temperature setting to 350 degrees Fahrenheit (176.7 degrees Celsius) to preheat.
2. Mix the sunflower and pumpkin seeds, ground flax, maca root and dried currants in a large bowl. Make sure that the ingredients are well distributed and that no large clumps of any ingredient can be seen.
3. Mix the melted coconut oil, sweetener, and salt and spices in a small bowl. Make sure that the ingredients are carefully mixed as well.
4. Pour the bowl of liquid into the mixture of seeds then mix. Make sure that all of the seed mixture is uniformly coated.
5. Using parchment paper, cover the baking sheet that will be used for the mixture. Ensure the uniform distribution and stability of the paper to avoid messy outcomes. Spread the resulting mixture evenly onto the baking sheet. Let it stay inside the oven for 10 minutes.
6. Carefully take out the baking sheet and then make sure that the mixture is evenly distributed on the sheet. Place it back in the oven. This step will prevent the mixture from burning.
7. Repeat step 7 at a 10- or 15-minute interval. Continue the procedure until the mixture is baked for a total of 35 to 40 minutes.
8. Cool the resulting product for about 30 minutes. This cereal, among other **Grain**

free Recipes, is best served with yoghurt and fruits.

Grain free Recipes can be quite a turning point for people who are used to consuming ordinary cereals and legumes in their everyday diet. Nonetheless, a change in one's nutrition plan can suggest rather more advantages provided that a dieter will observe proper food preparation.

Simple Grain Free Recipes: A Different Side Of Pancakes

Ready-to-cook pancakes that can be found in any local grocery store may be a bit of a risk both to dieters who do not wish to consume grains and those who are allergic to grains. This is because of the possibility that grains may be present in any product offered in the market. Thus, **Grain free Recipes**, like the one discussed below, are necessary for satisfying the needs of these dieters.

Engaging in a diet plan different from the ordinary requires not only the will to sacrifice the usual meals one enjoys but also the patience in coming up with items that comply with the demands of the plan. Specifically, **Grain free Recipes**, as what the name suggests, are composed of some ingredients that may not be readily available in the market. To comply with the demands of this kind of diet, a dieter may be obliged to provide substitute ingredients that can ensure a grain-free dish. For example, this dish includes almond flour since the commercial flour sold in local grocery stores usually contains grain products. In addition, per 125 grams of almond flour, there is only a calorie intake of 180. There is also a negligible presence of cholesterol, let alone sodium and sugar. This is because generally, almonds are one of the best known healthy nuts. They contain low calories and provide support for the heart.

Consequently, producing ingredients from commodities that can be found in the kitchen may also be necessary because of the need of substitute items in making **Grain free Recipes**. In this matter, baking powder is preferred to be homemade to ensure that it really is grain-free. If, however, there are ready-made products in the grocery store that claim such, it is alright to prefer using them since it will be much easier.

This is one of the easiest **Grain free Recipes** available for those who wish to pursue this diet. However, like other **Grain free Recipes**, it still requires work in other parts, such as assuring that all the ingredients to be used do not contain grains.

These are the ingredients for one of the numerous **Grain free Recipes**:

- ✓ 1/4 teaspoon of almond extract
- ✓ 1/4 teaspoon of unflavored gelatin (optional)*
- ✓ 1/2 teaspoon of baking soda
- ✓ 1/2 teaspoon of grain-free baking powder
- ✓ 2 teaspoons of raw honey
- ✓ 2 tablespoons of coconut flour
- ✓ 1/2 cup of almond flour
- ✓ 1/2 cup of full fat cottage cheese
- ✓ 3 eggs
- ✓ a pinch of salt
- ✓ coconut oil
- ✓ butter

✓ honey or maple syrup

*The job of gelatin is to make a sturdier mixture that will not create too much mess when put in the skillet.

The following utensils which may also be needed in other **Grain free Recipes** are required for use in creating these pancakes.

✓ Bowl
✓ food processor or mixer
✓ skillet

To make the pancakes, this process has to be followed. Fortunately, unlike other **Grain free Recipes**, it does not require that much time and work in the procedure.

1. Put all the ingredients (except the last three ones) in a bowl. Using a food processor or mixer, carefully mix the ingredients until smooth and no large clumps is visible.
2. Heat a large skillet using medium setting. Drop some coconut oil and move the skillet in such a manner that the oil will be evenly distributed.
3. Check if the skillet is hot enough by placing one palm above the skillet. When enough heat is acquired, place spoonfuls of the batter in the skillet. The size and number of the pancakes will depend on the amount of batter in every serving.
4. Let the batter cook until the bottom side is golden brown and bubbles forming on top start to pop. When this happens, flip the

pancakes and wait until the other side is cooked.

5. Repeat steps 3 and 4, constantly putting coconut oil after every batch, until all the batter has been cooked.

6. Place pancakes in a plate and put a cube of butter on top. Drizzle with honey or maple syrup if desired.

This is perfect for breakfast, although it can be served at any time of the day. Dieting should not be a challenge since **Grain free Recipes** do not necessarily need to be difficult to make especially with ingredients that can be found at home.

www.ingramcontent.com/pod-product-compliance
Lightning Source LLC
Chambersburg PA
CBHW070255290526
45789CB00004B/1858